NATURAL TIPS FOR STAYING HEALTHY

DURING THE 2020 PANDEMIC AND BEYOND

ANN MUSICO,

CERTIFIED HOLISTIC HEALTH
AND WHOLENESS COACH

CONTENTS

DEAR HEALTH SEEKER:

I put this book together with the best information I was able to find for how to protect against COVID-19.

As a holistic health and wholeness coach, I believe in doing things in the most natural way and I prefer to strengthen my own immune system and work on prevention rather than dealing with healing from something, including this virus.

I did a series of newsletters when this all began and so this is what you have here, all the newsletters, plus a page where I share some of the strategies I've been using on a daily and weekly basis to stay healthy, my personal protocol. It is shared for information purposes only, to give you an idea of things you may consider adding into your routines.

My prayer is that some of the ideas will be helpful for you and your family and that you stay healthy and strong, during this pandemic and beyond.

You can sign up for my newsletter at: https://www.threedimensionalvitality.com/Free_Newsletter.html

I will put links to those resources, blogs, newsletters, research and articles mentioned at the end of the book for your convenience.

Ann

Dear Health Seeker:

The information provided in this book is designed to provide helpful information on the subjects discussed. This book is not meant to be used, nor should it be used, to diagnose or treat any medical condition. For diagnosis or treatment of any medical problem, consult your own physician. The publisher and author are not responsible for any specific health or allergy needs that may require medical supervision and are not liable for any damages or negative consequences from any treatment, action, application or preparation, to any person reading or following the information in this book. References are provided for informational purposes only and do not constitute endorsement of any websites or other sources. Readers should be aware that the websites listed in this book may change.

PROACTIVE HEALTH PRACTICES

The definition of being proactive is "creating or controlling a situation by causing something to happen rather than responding to it after it has happened." In light of the Coronavirus, which we are and have been experiencing, it clarifies the two choices we always have when it comes to our health: we can be proactive or reactive.

Clearly being proactive is the preferred choice for many reasons. Studies show that being proactive about your health not only results in better health care; it also strengthens your body's natural self-repair mechanisms and helps your body fend off illness. When we take the time and put the effort in to establishing habits that support our overall health and well-being, when there is a crisis, we are much better able to deal with it.

Whenever it is a health crisis that affects a large number of people, it's always true that we hear conflicting information and the whole truth is only revealed over time. But what are we to do in the meantime? Perhaps we can look at this particular crisis as a wake-up call. If you were caught unprepared this time, why not make the decision that you will not let that happen again?

Everything you do begins with a thought and a decision. Has this crisis convinced you that being prepared and changing your habits is worth the effort? If so, I applaud you. I want to set forth some ideas, thoughts and strategies you may choose to implement and make part of your daily routines and habits. Choose those that you feel would make the biggest impact on your overall health.

You don't have to incorporate them all. Identify the areas you feel could be strengthened and take several weeks or months to begin adding in some strategic habits that will address areas you feel are weakest. What follows is an overview of the general areas you may want to consider beefing up so to speak.

Habits or Genes?

While this Coronavirus crisis has to do with an outside pathogen, **a virus**, all too often we slip into lazy, unhealthy habits and before you know it, may begin experiencing the beginnings of chronic disease. It is easier, I know, to just blame it all on our genes, but that excuse has been debunked.

There are certainly genetic propensities for certain diseases. For instance cancer runs in my family. The majority of my ancestors died from that awful disease. While I am aware, I also know it doesn't mean I have to develop that disease – or any disease.

Enter epigenetics. This prefix, 'epi,' comes from the Greek for 'over, on top of'. Therefore, epigenetics is an additional layer of instructions that lies 'on top of' DNA, controlling how our genes are read, interpreted and expressed. These are external modifications to DNA that turn genes "on" or "off." These changes do not change the actual DNA sequence, but instead, affect how cells "read" genes.

By incorporating certain habits, we can affect which genes are expressed and which are silenced. That's huge and so powerful and such good news! Where you may have felt you were a victim of your genes, this puts the power back in your hands. Diet and other external environmental influences can potentially play a role in controlling epigenetic processes.

Best Practices

I can't imagine anyone arguing the point that the best way to stay healthy is to prevent problems from developing in the first place. Prevention is SO much easier than correction. For example, making changes to your diet and habits when you are made aware that you have developed pre-diabetes is easier than waiting until you have full blown diabetes and then back pedaling and trying to reverse it. It's not impossible, it's just much more difficult.

The hard, sad truth is: many diseases and conditions are the result of poor choices that accumulate over the course of many years. Every day, millions of Americans deal with the effects of chronic disease. According to the CDC, the disturbing statistics are that 6 in 10 U.S. adults have a chronic disease and 4 in 10 have at least two chronic diseases!

We now have so many tools available to us in order to monitor different conditions, including pedometers, heart rate monitors, fitness trackers, more sensitive and specific blood tests, glucose monitors, apps and other tools. Using these and other tools, we can check what's going on and adjust our activities accordingly. So the first step is making the decision to become proactive.

Make the quality decision that you will commit to making whatever changes necessary, gradually, but definitely and consistently. Just as a health crisis or chronic disease can be a huge catalyst of positive change in your life, it's all in the way you choose to frame it and respond to it.

How prepared you are going into any crisis makes a difference in how successfully you will navigate it and come through. So I encourage you to think calmly, soberly and honestly about areas you may need to make changes in. Pray about those changes and assess whether you truly are ready to take some specific steps to put yourself in a more positive position.

FOUNDATIONAL FOODS AND SUPPLEMENTS

What are the Basics:

Food is or should be your first course of action for health and healing. We all eat every day! So choosing the healthiest, highest quality, real foods to keep yourself strong should be step one. We are talking about being proactive and putting habits in place to protect you should another crisis arise. I will just reiterate what I believe are the basics of healthy eating and then share my thoughts on things to keep on hand for those times someone is under the weather (like cold and flu season that comes every year) or some health crisis arises.

I will begin with the basics:

First, choose high quality food. This means organic, grass-fed/finished, wild caught and pasture raised.

Second, choose one-ingredient foods in a form as close to how God made them as possible. So, choose foods that *are* ingredients as opposed to those that have in-gredients. For example, chicken, lamb, mushrooms, salmon, rice, cucumbers, apples, broccoli, raspberries, walnuts. You get the idea.

Finally, choose those foods that agree with your particular metabolic makeup. The first two are pretty easy to understand. However, no matter how healthy a particular food is, if you are sensitive to it, it doesn't agree with you or you just plain do not like it – don't eat it!

Besides being fuel, food is meant to be enjoyed. Choosing those high quality, one-ingredient foods is the basic blueprint when it comes to food. So fresh and frozen organic veggies and fruits should be in your fridge and freezer all the time, along with properly raised animal products.

What about Water

Before I move on to things you can have on hand, let's just highlight the importance of drinking clean, pure water. I am on a well at my house and it is very high in sulfur. We began using bottled, distilled water when we first moved into our house and found that my youngest son was highly allergic to the sulfur in the water. So I still use distilled water, to which I add **trace minerals**.

Staying hydrated at all times just keeps all your body systems functioning optimally. When trying to avoid a virus or illness or get over one, hydration is even more critical. Also drinking unsweetened teas and coffee offer antioxidants and polyphenols. EGCG, an antioxidant in green tea is known to be a potent anti-viral.

According to Pique Tea, despite a perpetual myth that caffeinated tea is dehydrating, repeated studies show no difference in hydration levels between those who drink water and those who drink tea. This applies to caffeinated teas also. While caffeine is a diuretic, you'd have to drink about 10 cups of tea to experience a diuretic effect.

That being said, the bulk of your hydration should come from clean water.

One other thing I do is that I write "Love and Gratitude" on the water containers. I do this for a good reason which I explain in more detail in Today is Still the Day on page 146. Briefly, in accordance with the research of Dr. Masaru Emoto on how water responds to both written and spoken words, I choose to use words of love, blessing and gratitude wherever I can, including on my water!

Supplements and Supplemental Food Products:

Before I get into the foods to stock up on, I need to highlight the importance of eliminating added sugar from all sources. Sugar depresses the immune system. This is the opposite of what you want. You can use natural sweeteners like stevia, erythritol and Lakanto to sweeten your beverages or any healthy treats you make.

But I urge you to eliminate packaged, processed, sugary "treats" – cookies, cakes, cereals, crackers, candy, muffins, soda (including artificially sweetened sodas) and at least limit processed grain consumption since they are quickly converted to sugar in the body. What are some of the things I make sure I have on hand at all times that supplement my meals that are created from real, high quality foods?

I thought it would be easiest if I list food products and supplements separately and just give you the links. You can look at whatever interests you. ***Any product with an asterisk is one I sell and I receive a small commission.**

Food Products:

Green Powders – I alternate between these.
*Youngevity Super Greens

OrganiGreens

Collagen Broth

Bone Broth

Pu'erh and Reishi Mushroom Teas Life Extension published research showing that reishi mushroom and pu-erh tea extracts support immune cell health, response and ratio. While they have a supplement that includes these as well as other ingredients, I find it easiest to include a sachet of each of these once a week or so in my morning elixir.

Coconut Oil Coconut oil is high in lauric acid which forms monolaurin when digested and can kill harmful pathogens, such as bacteria, viruses, and fungi. (See Lauricidin below). I cook with it and even take a teaspoon or two straight if I feel a scratchy throat coming on.

I also use it to oil pull every morning. By keeping your teeth and gums clean you protect your immune system as well. It's a win-win.

Manuka Honey More powerful than regular honey. Another one I use as soon as I feel a scratchy throat.

Flax Seeds I include a scoop in my smoothies and daily green drink. You can also include it in baked goods. The lignans are very protective, it is a good source of fiber, antioxidants and omega 3s. It is a wonderful food to nourish the immune system.

Beef Sticks

Turkey Sticks

Protein Powders – I switch around so always have several different ones available. I mix a scoop of powder in a liquid of my choice and shake up for a quick hit of nutrition or I include a scoop in a protein smoothie with greens, berries and other foods to make a more substantial meal replacement.

***Youngevity Collagen Peptides**

***Slender FX Meal Replacement Shake**

***TMR Total Meal Replacement Shake**

***Youngevity FitShake**

*True Keto Shake

Supplements:

Vitamin C. It's important to know that many hospitals are using vitamn C for extremely sick patients. I regularly take 4,000 mg daily and if I feel a cold coming on, I double that or more.

Vitamin D3

***Selenium**

Quercetin

Zinc lozenges

Manuka Honey and Propolis lozenges

Melatonin and **Tryptophan** - Here is some **interesting research** about how these may affect healing.

Probiotics – We use a rotation strategy, alternating between a few different trusted brands (with different strains and species). You can also take different brands on alternate days to help increase microbial diversity.

Vitacost probiotic

Organixx Probiotixx

Just Thrive Probiotic

Enzymes – we take with meals to more fully get the benefits of the nutrition and between meals on an empty stomach (particularly protease) to scavenge viruses and other bugs:

Organixx P3E

R-Garden Protease

***Colloidal Silver**

Iodine – we alternate between these two:

Vitacost Kelp

Survival Shield Nascent Iodine

***Beta Glucan RVB 300**

NAC

Medicinal mushrooms (besides my mushroom coffee!) This goes in green drinks and smoothies.

Lauricidin I get this from my chiropractor but if you can't, you can order online. We started using it when my husband was bitten by a tick and had some bad side effects from the antibiotic and medication the doctor gave him. It is natural and very effective to protect you from viruses as well.

Senolytic Activator Senescent (aging) cells can accumulate over time, affecting the day-to-day function of the healthy cells around them. Senolytic compounds selectively target senescent cells. My husband and I take this supplement once a week as we are in that higher risk age group and cells naturally age.

<u>Final Words</u>: Obviously I don't take all these things every day! I do take many regularly, but they are also some of the things I depend on when it's **cold and flu season** or during a crisis like the one we just experienced. It pays to have your pantry stocked with foods and supplements you can use when you may not be able to get out to the stores or they may not have a full supply.

SPIRIT AND SOUL

If you truly want to be proactive about your health, you must include other aspects of your life as well as diet. Before I focus on spiritual and soul health, I wanted to also remind you that adequate, restful sleep is critical to staying healthy – at all times! When you are sleep deprived, it depresses your immune function.

Please do whatever you need to in order to have restful, rejuvenating sleep. Make your bedroom conducive to rest and relaxation; avoid blue light and anything stimulating close to bedtime; try to make your last meal at least 3 hours before bedtime; use natural supplements if you need some help like tryptophan, melatonin, CBD and magnesium.

Why it's Healthy:

Emotional and mental distress and anxiety can be as much of a contributor to health conditions as bad eating habits and lack of physical activity are, and some research even suggests that loneliness can be worse for our health than smoking. In fact experts believe diet, nutrition and health habits account for 20% of risk of developing chronic diseases, and emotional health accounts for 80%.

Clearly we cannot afford to overlook this aspect of health. I want to share some of my thoughts and strategies for addressing the spiritual and soul aspects of dealing with any crisis and particularly a health crisis. So, as I do with all things, I begin with spirit because that is the real you. You are a spirit. You have a soul – a mind, will and emotions. You live in a physical body. I have said this many times before but I will reiterate it here just for the sake of clarity.

I am a Christian and I approach everything from my faith in God. I share my faith freely but I do not force my beliefs on anyone. So for me prayer, reading and studying the Bible, meditating on scripture and speaking faith confessions is the first step. Activate your faith, whatever that looks like for you.

I mentioned already, I write the words "love and gratitude" on my water containers. I also pray over my meals. I know there is power in our words and in our thoughts and there is great power in sincere, believing prayer.

According to Dr. Caroline Leaf: *thoughts have a physical structure and influence the production of bio-chemicals in our bodies. Thinking determines how you function spiritually, emotionally, mentally and physically. Every thought has a corresponding electrochemical reaction. Depending on the type of thought, specific bio-chemicals are released in response. Happiness, gratitude and love release certain chemicals and sadness, anger and fear release different ones. Thoughts have the power to change your whole system. (As a man thinks so is he! Pr. 23:7)*

Dr. Joseph Prince says this and I think it beautifully summarizes the interplay and importance of beliefs, thoughts, words and emotions:

"You see, people are struggling to control their behaviors and actions because they don't have control over their emotions and feelings. They don't have control over their emotions and feelings because they don't have control over their thoughts. And they don't have control over their thoughts because they are not controlling what they believe."

Forgiveness and Gratitude

I must touch on two things that are critically important and relate to both spirit and soul, which often overlap: Forgiveness and Gratitude.

Walking in love and forgiveness is a basic tenet of my faith. They are also powerful immune boosters. A few documented health benefits of forgiveness, besides boosting immune function, include improved mental health, lower blood pressure, fewer symptoms of depression, less anxiety, stress and hostility, and improved cardiovascular health. It's been said refusing to forgive is like taking poison and expecting the other person to die.

I encourage you to forgive for your own benefit. It doesn't mean you have to like the person or trust them. Just release yourself from the bondage of unforgiveness.

Something powerful I want to share about anger is that in Ephesians 4:26 NLT we are told: And "don't sin by letting anger control you. Don't let the sun go down while you are still angry." In meditating on this scripture I felt the Lord highlighted a reason I hadn't ever seen in quite this way. When we sleep our bodies go through certain cleaning and restorative functions throughout the night. If we go to sleep angry, our bodies continue to release stress hormones and short-circuit this very powerful and critical function.

Gratitude is extremely powerful. I have written blog posts in the past about the benefits and I share them below:

Health and Longevity: More Gratitude Benefits

Brain Health: Why Gratitude is Powerful

Health Benefits of Gratitude

I have an interesting little experiment you can try. I call it **"The Good Old Days"** exercise and I believe it is very relevant for such a time as this.

Soul Strategies

Let's start with the mind – thinking. I mentioned above what Dr. Caroline Leaf says about the power in our thoughts. What if we begin being much more careful and intentional about what we allow into our minds through what we watch, read and listen to? I believe it will go a very long way toward moving us from negativity to positivity (which has health benefits all its own) and from fear, anxiety and worry to peace, joy and love.

You have ultimate control over the programs and videos you watch, the music and podcasts you listen to and the books, articles and posts you read. I propose you guard your mind and reject negative health beliefs as well. Just because your doctor or some health expert says there's only a 10% chance you'll recover, doesn't mean you have to think like a pessimist and look at the glass as 90% empty. Reframe those numbers and focus on the fact that 10% of people with your disease get well – and for the 10% who do, the other 90% don't matter.

It's important to realize that positive health outcomes aren't just flukes. Those who get well against all odds share these common proactive characteristics.

Your will is important in that the strength of your convictions, your commitment and consistency depend on the strength and health of your will. I talk about Complete Hydration in Today is Still the Day as it relates to spirit, soul and body. When your will is parched you become paralyzed and can't make a decision. You never want your will to become dry, brittle and tired. There is a fine line between exercising it (like any muscle it needs exercise to grow) and resting it so it doesn't become fatigued.

Putting routines in place and preparing ahead allow you to automate daily habits so you don't have to constantly be making decisions. Your spirit and soul definitely overlap when it comes to your emotions, and even your body in some ways. For example, if you are dehydrated, you cannot properly process emotions. Eating large amounts of typical, high sugar comfort foods causes spikes and dips in blood sugar that cause emotional instability as well insulin resistance. Besides what I have already mentioned, there are some other things you might consider in order to maintain your emotional stability and serenity regardless of what is going on around you.

Spending time in nature is a wonderful way to reboot your emotions as well as lowering cortisol, pulse rate and blood pressure, increasing parasympathetic nerve activity, lowering sympathetic nerve activity as well as boosting the immune system by increasing activity of natural killer cells. I have written blog posts about the benefits of spending time outdoors and you can read them below.

Health and Stress: Nature is a Natural Stress Reducer

Health and Wholeness: Getting Back to Nature

Health: The Nature Prescription

Another, perhaps unique, but very effective strategy is grounding or earthing. Simply walking barefoot in the grass or on the sand of the beach reconnects you to the earth's anti-inflammatory, antioxidant electrons. It has been found to decrease inflammation in your body, which can help quiet down back pain and other types of pain; improve energy, reduce anxiety and stress, improve sleep, cardiovascular function and hormonal cycles. Your immune system functions optimally when your body has an adequate supply of negatively charged electrons, which are easily and naturally obtained by barefoot/bare skin contact with the earth.

You can also purchase bands, sheets and mats online. I use a band that I put on my wrist when I am sitting down in the evening and ground for several hours before bedtime. I highly recommend it.

Practicing EFT, particularly, in the moment when you are experiencing fear, anxiety or stress is an exceptionally simple, yet effective way to go beyond just managing stress.

Something you may not have thought about doing is **coloring in an adult coloring book**. There are so many really beautiful ones out there — some with bible verses, others with pictures of butterflies, flowers and nature or just uplifting quotations. The act of sitting quietly and coloring has been proven to rank right up there with meditation in its ability to calm anxiety.

Of course music is always powerful as it bypasses the conscious mind. Choosing music you love but that will be uplifting and calming is key. Also listening to nature sounds like birds chirping, a babbling brook or rainstorm are also very relaxing. I have CDs of those sounds and listen to them often as well as to other music, including **Wholetones**, that I truly love and enjoy.

Of course staying active on a daily basis is helpful in so many ways, not the least of which is releasing feel good endorphins.

Final Words:

I hope these suggestions will be helpful to you and that you will begin implementing some of them in your regular, normal routine so that you will be prepared should another crisis occur. All this negativity surrounding us brings our vibration DOWN. We become fearful, anxious with the potential of becoming depressed. DON'T even go there. We create our own reality. We are not victims.

This is a hard one in times like this when we are being brutally forced into thinking like victims. Is it deliberate? Fear is a great control mechanism. Whether we allow ourselves to be fearful is up to us. Ultimately, we have control over ourselves, what we feel, what we think. That's incredibly powerful. As energetic beings keeping energetically positive will raise our vibrations. This of course will keep us well balanced and healthy.

TOP TWO RISK FACTORS

We heard that the populations most at risk for contracting the virus and being hospitalized are those with underlying health conditions and the elderly. "Elderly" is considered to be anyone 60 and above. I take offense to being called elderly at my age! I don't expect that description until I am 90, so I have quite a ways to go.

Several studies found that people's level of satisfaction with their relationships at age 50 was a better predictor of physical health than their cholesterol levels were. By the way, those people with the lowest LDL cholesterol levels were found to have the highest risk of contracting COVID. Totally opposite of what mainstream medicine tells us about cholesterol but that's a different subject.

The people who were the most satisfied in their relationships at age 50 were the healthiest at age 80. Perhaps we should spend a little more time on building satisfying, loving relationships and less time worrying about the details. Just a thought.

That being said, I want to talk about two important factors and how you can begin now to improve your health and immune function before the next "novel" virus or some other health crisis comes around.

#1 Risk Factor – Age

Let's begin with the #1 risk factor, age. There is such a thing as immune senescence, or age-related immune impairment. Despite a healthy lifestyle, aging often seems to be accompanied by declines in immune function. More serious complications and deaths occur in older people compared to younger people with more vibrant immune function.

Let me say that one reason is that older people are more likely to be on medications and managing other underlying, chronic diseases. However, this issue of immune impairment can affect even healthy older adults. This is also why vaccines often fail in older people - because of their inability to generate a strong enough antibody response. This runs contrary to the recommendations for older people to be sure to get flu and pneumonia vaccines we hear about every year. So what can we do? Are we just out of luck? Not at all!!

If you go back to the section on food and supplements you will see there are many natural, effective vitamins and supplements, including vitamins C, D, zinc, magnesium, melatonin, garlic, and quercetin and the Senolytic Activator to name a few.

The other thing I want to share with you is something I practice personally and that is, the moment I feel the very beginnings of a cold or any viral infection – a slightly dry, scratchy throat, for instance – I immediately begin to up my intake of these supplements. I take aggressive, proactive action and I can honestly say that it has never failed to stop a possible cold or flu before it ever took hold.

I eat well, practice intermittent fasting, hydrate well, exercise and stay active daily and get adequate sleep.

<u>My perspective is this</u>: I am blessed to still be here at 66. There is still much I want to do and I certainly want to fully enjoy my children and grandchildren. So proactively taking steps to ensure I remain strong and healthy for as long as I can is a no-brainer. I have been doing this for so many years it is just my normal way of life.

What I want people to realize is that they are not victims. Oh dear, I am "elderly" so I'm out of luck. NO!! There's plenty you can do including speaking positive health confessions over yourself and practicing gratitude. You are still here for a reason. God has a purpose for you, so take care of the amazing temple He fashioned for you to live in for as long as you are blessed to be here. If you need help specifically with this, **please don't hesitate to contact me**.

We may not be able to turn the clock back, but we can keep it running as well as possible by daily incorporating a few simple steps and being proactive.

#2 Risk Factor – Obesity

Some studies suggest that obesity is second only to age as a risk factor for hospitalization from COVID-19, *even when no other health conditions are present*. Obesity is increasingly linked to serious cases of COVID-19 that require hospitalization, even among young people.

Here are some numbers to consider:

Almost 70% of Americans are overweight and 40% are obese.

One in three has either pre-diabetes or diabetes and the #1 cause of death in this country is heart disease, which is linked to both obesity and **diabetes**.

So approximately half of Americans are at increased risk of complications due to COVID-19 and perhaps any other viral infection that appears in the future!

What is very important to realize is this and please don't miss it:

<u>Most of the pre-existing conditions that increase the risk of morbidity and mortality from COVID-19 or other viruses are impacted by diet and lifestyle, and are completely preventable.</u>

Again – if you are overweight, obese or have been diagnosed with pre-diabetes or diabetes – you are not a victim. There are powerful, effective steps you can take to improve your health right now. Let's focus in on obesity and why this is such a big risk factor and how you can empower yourself.

Visceral fat, the deep, internal fat that surrounds your organs, is extremely active. It is constantly creating inflammatory chemicals and releasing them into your body. This is especially dangerous because the biggest offender in this virus is the cytokine storm that can overwhelm your body with inflammatory molecules. If you're already chronically inflamed, this cytokine storm can hit you even harder.

In a nutshell, here are the other reasons carrying excess weight is dangerous in this situation:

Overweight or obese people shed more virus particles and shed them for a longer time, endangering others;

Hospitalized patients are also more likely to develop secondary infections.

The bottom line is that excess weight causes inflammation and increases risk of type 2 diabetes. Infections are more common and often more serious in diabetics because **high blood sugar levels** cause the body to produce molecules that weaken its infection-fighting defenses.

If you are overweight or obese right now, I know all this sounds like really bad news. But that's not the end of the story. Instead of focusing on the negative and what we can't do, let's focus on **what we can do.**

There is also very good news: every pound you lose right now will improve your immune function and help to protect you against COVID-19 and other viral infections.

One study shows that even a small amount of weight loss starts to reverse immune system damage. The authors of one study found that simply losing about 13 pounds was enough to "bring the pro-inflammatory nature of circulating immune cells back to that found in lean people." This means that you can begin healing your immune system very quickly.

Every pound you lose now will improve your immune function and protect you against COVID-19 and any other viral outbreaks you encounter in the future. And, unfortunately, you can be sure that there will be others.

MAKING CHANGES

Even during the best of times, building new daily habits is challenging and replacing bad habits with good ones can be even more difficult.

If this experience has taught us anything, I believe it is that adopting healthier habits is even more important than ever. Regardless of your health status, this just becomes even more critical.

Making these behavior changes becomes a bit more challenging given that we have limited access to not only grocery stores and gyms, but also to certain foods. Add to that the additional stressors, including loneliness and isolation many are facing and it could seem overwhelming.

<u>While there is no known drug or medication that "kills" a virus</u>, there are nutraceuticals that have an effect on them and support the immune system, while others have the ability to reduce your viral load.

Where Should We Focus?

So, instead of focusing on the so-called silver bullet (medication, vaccine) that "kills" the virus (which doesn't exist) or whatever the disease is, my suggestion is that we focus on the host instead. If the host (you, me) has a strong immune system,

he/she should be able to recover from COVID-19 and any other virus and receive immunity.

Remember, there are over 200 flu-like viruses with COVID-19 being only one of them. In the future, there will be other viruses and some may be more severe. We should be focusing on how to improve our health in order to give us the best chance to fight off a future infection.

Resetting, rejuvenating, supporting and rebooting our immune system function is, in my opinion, the best way to approach the future. There are many things we can do to accomplish this. Some were mentioned above and I will go into more detail about some others.

Focusing on what we can do, strengthening our body and supporting our immune system, rather than managing symptoms and treating the infectious organism is empowering! We have more power than we realize. Our bodies are Intelligently created with these amazing, built-in immune systems. We can strengthen them by what, when and how much we eat, managing stress, getting adequate sleep and exercise. All of these things influence how well our bodies respond to infection from any virus or bacteria.

Do An Inventory

My recommendation is that you consider the areas of your lifestyle that could be improved. Is it your diet? Getting enough sleep? Managing stress and fear? Incorporating exercise? You are not a powerless victim by any means.

Your body was created to heal itself *if* you provide the right raw materials. So let's talk about some of these things we can all address.

Oral Health and Immunity

I wanted to take a slightly different approach you may not have considered. While most of your immune system resides in your gut, it actually begins in your mouth! Your mouth has its own specific microbiome which is extremely important in your defense against this and any virus. Without a healthy mouth, you have a breeding ground for viruses and bacteria!

Here's why: everything that passes through your body, generally comes through your mouth first. The food you eat, the liquids you drink, medicines, allergens and more come through your mouth. It's not surprising that your oral health is strongly connected to your immune system function. If you have better oral health, you can expect to have better overall health and fewer illnesses.

There is a strong connection between your oral health and overall health, and scientists are finding more connections all the time. If left unchecked, bacteria in your mouth can affect many different systems in the body. Chronic inflammation and poor oral health has been linked to developing illnesses like heart disease, type 2 diabetes, lung conditions and Alzheimer's. Certain bacteria in your mouth can be pulled into your lungs, causing pneumonia and other respiratory diseases.

Dr. Mercola shared recent research linking certain mouthwashes possibly destroying the lipid layer of coronaviruses and preventing them from replicating in the throat. You can **read what he says here.** While those mouthwashes may be helpful for preventing COVID-19 they destroy healthy oral microbiome. It was also found later that these mouthwashes raised blood pressure, which is a risk factor. He does mention that oil pulling is a good alternative and one I recommend and practice daily.

Think about it. Your mouth is the perfect environment for bacteria to thrive. It's moist, warm, and usually has lots of nutrients for the bacteria to feed on. Food particles left in your mouth help bacteria grow; that's why it's so important to brush and floss daily. When bacteria grow out of control, they can cause both gum disease and tooth decay. As these conditions worsen, bacteria move from the mouth into the rest of the body. Bacteria from your mouth get into your bloodstream by way of diseased gums or places where teeth are damaged or missing setting off an immune response in the body.

C-reactive protein, or CRP, an inflammatory marker, is released from the liver. In the short term, it is a natural and appropriate response and doesn't do any harm, but if CRP is being released constantly (possibly due to bacteria in the mouth causing inflammation), then it can set off a chain reaction that eventually leads to other health conditions. I have already mentioned how underlying conditions like type 2 diabetes can compromise your immune function. Poor oral health is **very often linked with diabetes**.

I went into more detail about oral health in this past newsletter and shared some of my favorite resources and products.

Sleep and Your Immune System

Adequate, restful sleep is especially important right now to support a healthy and balanced immune response. It's always important, but it becomes even more critical during times of viral outbreaks. Every bodily function is based on our 24 hour circadian rhythm. Our sleep-wake cycle is part of this and is regulated by light and darkness and is directly connected to our immune function.

Here's how it works: At night when it gets dark, there's a drop in our stress hormone cortisol, along with other hormones from our sympathetic nervous system like epinephrine and norepinephrine, while hormones like melatonin, connected to immune function, increases during sleep. Immune system cells can also focus all efforts and energy on a strong attack against viruses and bacteria while you sleep.

Studies have proven that sleep deprivation makes you **more susceptible to the common cold**, so it stands to reason that it would compromise your ability to fight off other viruses as well. Lack of restful sleep is also linked to elevated blood pressure, known to be an underlying condition that influences how well you can deal with viral infections.

According to Matthew Walker, Ph.D., sleep scientist and author of Why We Sleep—Unlocking the Power of Sleep and Dreams, *"after just one night of only four to five hours of sleep, your natural killer cells—a main player in viral killing—drop by 70%."* There is an entire chapter in Today is Still the Day devoted to sleep and rest because it is also critical for successful weight loss. Three of the best, safest supplements I can recommend are magnesium (glycinate or threonate), melatonin and the amino acid l-tryptophan. Not coincidentally, you'll remember they are included in the supplements recommended for fighting viruses listed previously.

CHIROPRACTIC AND IMMUNE FUNCTION

I am a huge proponent of regular chiropractic care. I rarely miss my monthly appointment and one of my dearest friends and mentor is a chiropractor.

According to a 26-page report released on March 28, 2020:

"Considerable evidence has mounted to support active communication between the nervous system and the immune system. The nervous system, including the brain and the peripheral divisions can either stimulate or inhibit various activities of both the innate and adaptive immune systems. Chiropractic is a health care discipline which emphasizes the inherent recuperative power of the body to heal itself without the use of drugs or surgery. The practice of chiropractic focuses on the relationship between structure (primarily the spine) and function (as coordinated by the nervous system) and how that relationship affects the preservation and restoration of health. It is founded upon the principle that the body's innate recuperative power is affected by and integrated through the nervous system."

Chiropractic adjustments have been shown to reduce subluxations and improve the body's ability to adapt and heal effectively. The results of a 3 year study found that chiropractic patients had 200% greater immune competence than those who did not receive chiropractic care. And this improvement did not diminish with age.

This also improves the body's ability to adapt to stress and perform at a higher level. Chiropractic adjustments to reduce subluxation help you to think and move with better speed and skill, which can make a huge difference in your ability to live in a state of thriving.

I am all for anything that addresses the body's innate ability to heal itself by gently bringing the systems back into alignment. That is what chiropractic does and I would highly recommend it as an addition to your basic health practices.

INTERMITTENT FASTING

The quality of the food you eat as well as how much you eat is important for weight management and overall health. Nutrition is foundational because the largest volume of chemicals your internal organs are exposed to come from your food! This is why I am constantly stressing the quality of the fuel you put into your body.

The most powerful weapon you currently have for fighting obesity, chronic illness and aging is a healthy diet.

You can scroll through any of the previous newsletters and get information on my recommendations for creating the healthiest fuel blend for you. Of course, if you would like personalized help in doing this, contact me and we can set up a free consultation to discuss how we can best move forward.

Before I get into the benefits of intermittent fasting for immune function, let me just give you the basics to consider when upgrading your diet in order to improve your health:

Avoid or severely limit sugar and processed grains which convert quickly to sugar as sugar depresses your immune system;

Avoid **ultraprocessed foods**, which I don't even actually consider food at all;

Choose high quality, whole, nutrient-dense foods in a form as close to how God created them; and

Be sure to avoid dehydration. My basic recipe is one-half your body weight in ounces of water and ¼ tsp of natural, unprocessed salt for every 32 oz. you drink.

Ok now that those basics are out of the way let's talk about meal timing – when you eat - and why it is important for your immune function.

Why it's Healthy:

Intermittent fasting is a strategy that involves fasting (not eating) for a period of time followed by a period of feasting (eating). Benefits of intermittent fasting include increased autophagy, cellular rejuvenation, improved immune system function, and genetic repair. It reduces inflammation and the risk of disease. Simply by reducing inflammation it increases and improves immune function.

Your body only has a certain amount of energy available that it diverts into functions such as digestion, (which is considered energy expensive), physical movement, immunity, cognition, etc. The continual need to digest food diverts energy away from these other critical areas, while fasting conserves energy for use with these other systems.

When you eat food (regardless of how clean and pure it is), your immune system is activated to protect you from any unwanted microorganisms within the food. It doesn't matter whether the food is raw or cooked as nothing is truly sterile. When your immune system is activated in order to attack newly ingested pathogens, it is using up its energy reserves that could be used for other activities.

Fasting frees these white blood cells up to destroy dormant infections and other problematic areas. Intermittent fasting is an effective regulator of the immune system as it controls the amount of inflammatory cytokines that are released in the body. Two major cytokines Interleukin-6 and Tumor Necrosis Factor Alpha promote an inflammatory response in the body. **Studies have shown** that fasting reduces the release of these inflammatory substances.

There are several different ways to incorporate intermittent fasting into your lifestyle. You already do it to a degree – you don't eat while you are sleeping – so that is fasting. You can gradually increase the fasting window in order to enjoy more of the benefits. I go into more detail about this in **Today is Still the Day**. Basically you can begin with 12 hour fasting and feasting windows. So in this example, if you finish dinner at 7 pm, you would not eat until at least 7 am the next morning.

Once you get comfortable doing that you can extend your fasting window. Try 13 hours fasting and an 11 hour eating window. Then move on to 14/10 and what I practice most often is 16/8. When we call it a "feasting window" it doesn't mean you eat for the entire 12 hours or whatever your window is. It just means you confine your eating only to that time period. This gives your body that break from digesting foods and allows important housecleaning functions (autophagy) to take place.

I would just advise you to listen to your body and pay attention to how you feel when trying different fasting windows and choose what works best for you.

Benefits and Specific Conditions:

So to recap: intermittent fasting seems to have an overall healing effect on the body by giving the digestive system a rest and concentrating your internal system energies toward stimulating repair and protection mechanisms. Other positive effects include:

· Improved immune regulation

· Increased stress resistance

· Reduced overall inflammation

· Increased energy efficiency

· Stimulation of autophagy

Secrets and Tips:

While you do not have to eat less, just less often, the quality of your food becomes even more critical. Choose immune-supporting, anti-inflammatory, nutrient-dense foods. Focus on organic greens including chard, kale, and spinach, vegetables, including cucumber, celery, and broccoli, herbs and spices including turmeric, ginger, basil, garlic and mint, low glycemic index fruits including lemons, limes, and berries, healthy fats including avocado, coconut oil, extra virgin olive oil, grass-fed butter, and ghee, clean protein including grass-fed beef, free-range poultry and eggs, wild-caught fish, fermented foods including kimchi, kombucha, miso, sauerkraut, and kefir, and medicinal mushrooms including reishi, cordyceps, and turkey tail.

GROUNDING FOR IMMUNE HEALTH

Grounding or earthing is a therapeutic technique that involves doing activities that "ground" or electrically reconnect you to the earth. The most recent scientific research **has explored grounding for inflammation, cardiovascular disease, muscle damage, chronic pain, and mood.**

According to this study, grounding affects the living matrix, which is the central connector between living cells. Electrical conductivity exists within the matrix that functions as an immune system defense, similar to antioxidants. It is believed that through grounding, the **natural defenses of the body can be restored.**

There are different types of grounding, all of which focus on reconnecting yourself to the earth, through either direct or indirect contact. One of the easiest ways to ground yourself to the earth is to walk barefoot whether on grass, sand, or even mud. Allowing your skin to touch the natural ground can provide you with grounding energy.

Lying on the grass or sand at the beach is another way to increase contact with the earth. Wading or swimming in a lake or the ocean is another wonderful way. If you are not able to walk barefoot or choose not to, there are grounding mats, straps, sheets, blankets and patches you can purchase and use. I have a grounding strap that I put around my wrist to ground myself when I am sitting down in the evening.

In recent years, inflammation has been recognized as the leading trigger of chronic pain and most major, chronic health disorders, including cardiovascular disease, diabetes, arthritis, Alzheimer's, and cancer. Inflammation sets our bodies on fire and earthing or grounding appears to extinguish the flames through the transfer of negatively-charged electrons from the surface of the Earth into the body where they neutralize positively-charged destructive free radicals involved in chronic inflammation.

The Earth's energy makes the ground beneath our feet an extremely effective and abundant antioxidant! And it's free. No pills, no prescriptions. All you have to do is reconnect. Ongoing research has found that chronic inflammation is a major factor in many of the most prevalent diseases in our country. Chronic inflammation sets off a cascade of disease-causing effects and has been linked to Alzheimer's disease, cancer, heart disease and diabetes. People with chronic inflammation have a much greater risk of developing a serious condition. So moderating this inflammatory response via grounding can bolster your hardworking immune system.

EXERCISE AND IMMUNE FUNCTION

According to **recent research**, regular exercise may also help prevent **acute respiratory distress syndrome (ARDS)**, a lethal complication and major cause of death among patients with COVID-19.

There is an antioxidant made inside your body called extracellular superoxide dismutase (EcSOD). This antioxidant, which protects tissues and prevents disease by eliminating free radicals, is made in and excreted from your muscles and circulates in your blood. EcSOD secretion is increased by exercising. According to research a decrease in EcSOD is seen in many diseases, including acute lung disease, ischemic heart disease and kidney failure. *Even just one exercise session has been shown to increase production of this powerful antioxidant.*

Regular exercise has numerous health benefits, with protection against this severe respiratory disease condition being just one. You don't have to go to the gym to exercise. I give many suggestions in **Today is Still the Day**. My husband, who is at the gym 7 days a week has used resistance bands as his form of exercise during gym closures along with our 4-6 mile walks on the local trails when weather has permitted.

I have always worked out at home so it hasn't been much different for me in that way. I use 10 minute HIIT DVD workouts, I get up every 30 or 40 minutes and do jumping jacks, high knees or some other form of movement throughout the day. I also regularly use the Nitric Oxide dump, mentioned in **Today is Still the Day**, on certain days. There are plenty of ways to exercise so there really is no excuse.

I talked about immunosenescence, which describes the natural changes our immune systems undergo due to aging. However, along with diet, exercise helps improve immunosenescence by slowing down the aging processes of both the innate and adaptive arms of your immune system. It improves the function of natural killer cells and white blood cells, which are part of your innate immune system.

HAPPINESS AND IMMUNE FUNCTION

We know, from many studies, that mental states such as fear, stress and anxiety **can negatively influence health. The field of study that investigates how our mental states affect our physiology is called psychoneuroimmunology. As early as 1964,** magazine editor **Norman Cousins, diagnosed with a life threatening autoimmune disease called ankylosing spondylitis, and given a 1 in 500 chance of recovery rejected his doctors' prognosis and embarked on his own program of happiness therapy. He credits this with triggering his dramatic recovery. He established the Cousins Center** to continue investigating **whether and how psychological factors really can keep people healthy.**

Professor at the Cousins Center, Steven Cole has published a series of studies suggesting that negative mental states such as stress and loneliness affect immune responses, impacting our ability to fight disease. The way we see the world could affect everything from our risk of chronic illnesses such as diabetes and heart disease to the progression of conditions such as HIV and cancer. These researchers are continuing their studies to understand how the immune system and nervous system interact.

Studies conducted during the 1980s and early 1990s revealed that the brain is directly wired to the immune system. Parts of the nervous system connect with immune-related organs such as the thymus and bone marrow. Immune cells have receptors for neurotransmitters, suggesting that the brain/nervous system and immune system communicate.

Studies have borne out that happy people (those with positive well-being) were more likely to eat a healthier diet and be physically active (both of which impact healthy immune function); tend to enjoy more **restful sleep**; and specifically help keep **immune function strong**; reducing the risk of developing colds and respiratory infections.

One study of about 300 healthy people looked at the risk of developing a cold after individuals were given a common cold virus via nasal drops. The least happy people were almost three times as likely to develop the common cold compared to their happier counterparts! So your emotional state is very powerful in supporting immune function.

HUMIDITY AND IMMUNE FUNCTION

Dr. Mercola did an in-depth article here about how the level of humidity affects the transmission of viruses. You can read the article in its entirety but I wanted to pull out a few important points here.

It's no secret that cold and flu season happens in the cooler and colder winter months where we get less sun exposure (vitamin D3) and also because we are stuck inside in our homes, the air is dry and humidity is low from our furnaces and heating systems. While neither extreme is good, (too high humidity levels can encourage mold growth), dry air and low humidity can increase feelings of being congested as sinus membranes dry out and become irritated, as well as dry, irritated eyes and skin.

Too high humidity can also trigger feelings of nasal congestion. So maintaining a **proper level of humidity** can help to reduce the rate of respiratory infections and allergies. While we've been forced to stay in our homes, I found this piece of information very interesting:

Scientists found the rate of infection with COVID-19 **rose in interior spaces**. Interestingly, the highest number of infections were spread in the home (79.9%) followed by transportation (34%), including planes, trains, cars and buses. This demonstrates the need to address the indoor spread of infection and perhaps raises questions about the validity of keeping people locked down in their homes.

Most experts recommend keeping the humidity level indoors at **40-60%** which is believed to help moisturize membranes and reduce the risk of infection. Besides purchasing and running a humidifier, you can also keep a pot of water simmering on the stove or set bowls of water around, which will improve humidity as they evaporate into the air. Just be sure to keep a humidifier clean to avoid encouraging mold, fungi and bacteria growth which all pose health problems of their own.

EMFS AND 5G

We are a collection of frequencies and since our bodies are designed to operate at specific levels and frequencies, by being surrounded by man-made electromagnetic frequencies (EMFs) that are a quadrillion times higher than the natural EMF environment of the Earth, it is no surprise that this could result in biological harm or damage.

Why it's Unhealthy:

The primary danger of EMFs and what causes the increased risk of developing chronic disease is mitochondrial damage triggered by formation of one of the most damaging types of reactive nitrogen species. Low-frequency microwave radiation opens your voltage-gated calcium channels (VGCCs) located in the outer membrane of your cells, allowing an abnormal influx of calcium ions into the cell, which in turn activates nitric oxide (NO) and superoxide, which react nearly instantaneously to form peroxynitrite, the damaging reactive nitrogen species.

By the way, just for your information, the highest density of VGCCs are found in your nervous system, brain, the pacemaker in your heart and in male testes. So it isn't difficult to believe that EMFs are likely to contribute to neurological and neuropsychiatric problems, heart and reproductive problems, including, among other things, cardiac arrhythmias, anxiety, depression, autism, Alzheimer's and infertility.

This results in massive oxidative stress by creating free radicals, which are associated with an increased level of systemic inflammation, mitochondrial dysfunction and DNA damage, thought to be a root cause for many of today's chronic diseases. Devices that continuously emit EMF radiation at levels that damage your mitochondria include your cellphone, cellphone towers, Wi-Fi routers and modems, baby monitors and "smart" devices of all kinds, including smart meters and smart appliances.

Also if you have a cell phone you wear on your wrist, use blue tooth technology or carry your cell phone on your person as I see some people do, you are being constantly exposed to close range EMF radiation.

EMFs of all types have been called an "invisible poison" we don't even know is affecting us. Some who are hypersensitive feel the effects ***but most of us do not*** until some area of our health breaks down. According to Russian studies, its effect on the gut brain axis causes over-stimulation of the vagus nerve resulting in disregulation of glucose metabolism which causes increase in diabetes, and structural alterations in vagus nerve synapses and communication.

Another well researched way in which EMF interacts with our bodies is through the pineal gland and melatonin reduction. Melatonin is responsible for regulating our sleep, for bodily repair functions, and preventing cancer. Our pineal glands make melatonin when it's dark. The problem with EMF is that the body can't tell the difference between it and light. Therefore, enough EMF in the bedroom will ensure that little melatonin is produced, resulting in insomnia. As I mentioned earlier, sleep deprivation makes you more susceptible to the common cold and other viruses.

I think you can at least agree that we are surrounded and inundated with these frequencies and they are definitely causing harm.

What is 5G:

So what is 5G anyway? "G" stands for Generation and refers to the frequency band it uses to receive and transmit data. 4G is 10 times faster than 3G and 5G is predicted to be 1000 times faster than our current systems. 5G is simply the fifth generation of mobile internet connectivity. It differs from the previous generations through its use of higher frequencies, which enable its users to transfer wireless data faster.

5G relies primarily on the **bandwidth of the millimeter wave (MMW)**, known to penetrate 1 to 2 millimeters of human skin tissue, causing a painful burning sensation. It's also been linked to eye and heart problems, **suppressed immune function**, genetic damage and fertility problems. This ability to penetrate tissue and cause a severe burning sensation is exactly why MMW was chosen for use in crowd control weapons (Active Denial Systems) by the U.S. Department of Defense.

5G is very real and is **making people very sick**. The frequencies being used for 5G are currently being used in weapons systems called active denial. Despite the intentional harm being caused by similar technology, there has been zero research done on the health effects of having 5G installed on a lamp post outside our homes – short or long term.

Is There any Connection to 5G and Immune Function:

Whether you believe that it is benign technology or not, rolling it out without the proper care or concern to our well-being is clearly unfair at best and oppressive and unjust at worst. 5G is now being commonly, **linked to COVID-19**. Numerous highly qualified and experienced doctors are describing the symptoms associated with 5G exposure as being very similar to those attributed to the virus.

Statistics also show a direct correlation between virus cases and 5G infrastructure. *EMF radiation from any and all sources adversely affects us. It over-works our immune systems which detect it as an attack in exactly the same way it does with viruses and bacteria.*

So, while our immune system is busy trying to eliminate something it can do nothing about (5G), it stops doing its job of eliminating the things it can and was intended to do something about – bacteria and viruses.

At the time of this writing, there are 58 cities in 32 states that have some form of 5G. Some states have only 1 provider while others have as many as four. The number of cities with 5G within each state also varies with California having the most cities (nine) with 5G at this writing.

<u>A weakened immune system is going to succumb more easily to any virus including the Coronavirus.</u> All of us have weakened immune systems to some degree because of our lifestyles, diet, age and habits and that includes our EMF exposure, but 5G weakens even the strongest among us as we can see by the spread of COVID–19 in Wuhan City, China, Italy, Spain and all the places where 5G was and is prevalent.

How Do You Protect Your Personal Environment:

There are many suggestions for how you can reduce your exposure to WIFI and 5G including keeping our cell phones on airplane mode when we are not using them, turning WIFI off in your home, especially at night while sleeping, using things like Faraday bags **for your cellphone, laptop and even router to shield yourself, painting your bedroom with shielding paint, plugging in a device in your home like a Stetzerizer or Greenwave filter that decrease the level of dirty electricity or electromagnetic interference being generated in your home and plenty of other options.**

Here's a 2-page 5G fact sheet you can look through at your leisure.

How Can You Protect Yourself:

This has been a huge concern for me. I know too many people who have been struggling for years with symptoms and have never gotten a definitive diagnosis. They've made every change possible and still have no resolution. People have been absolutely panic-stricken that there's an "invisible" virus floating around in the air that they must mask up to protect against.

Well this seems to me to be a much more insidious and devastating issue as it seems to be here to stay and the negative effects will only increase over time. I have been been researching this issue for several years and was introduced to wearable technology that has been thoroughly researched and tested to neutralize EMFs and 5G as well as optimizing cellular function and improving muscular strength. There are **compelling videos** with very credible information you will want to see.

I did my own research on this particular technology as I've used others over the years, and find this to be superior so in the interests of transparency I have not only purchased the bands for myself and my husband but I am also an affiliate. You may also order this protective wristband at this link.

I urge you to check out the information at the link and contact me about any questions.

I encourage and strongly urge you to take this danger seriously and to do your own research.

As a dear and respected friend so eloquently said, "The 5G protection device is analogous to wearing a bulletproof vest. The real solution is to be educated and vocal as 5G radiation becomes the silent bullet of destruction."

LYMPHATIC SYSTEM AND IMMUNE FUNCTION

The lymphatic system is like a network of highways that carries the garbage (waste, toxins, viruses, bacteria) out of your body. It is often overlooked and its importance underestimated. Its primary function is for immune function - to defend you against infection and disease. However it also allows fat-soluble vitamins like Vitamins A, D, E and K to get into your bloodstream and then throughout your body, as well as removing excess fluids from body tissues.

So what makes up your lymphatic system? It is a network of very small tubes (or vessels) that drain lymph fluid from all over the body. The major parts of the lymph tissue are located in the bone marrow, spleen, thymus gland, lymph nodes, and the tonsils. The heart, lungs, intestines, liver, bowels and skin also contain lymphatic tissue. Lymph nodes are round or kidney-shaped, and can be up to 1 inch in diameter. Most are found in clusters in the neck, armpit, and groin area as well as along the lymphatic pathways in the chest, abdomen, and pelvis, where they filter the blood.

While your circulatory system has a pump (your heart) to circulate your blood throughout all the miles of arteries and veins throughout your body, your lymphatic system does not have a pump. Your body actually has 3 times more lymph fluid than blood, but there is no organ to pump it. Physical movement and exercise, breathing, intestinal activity, and muscle action create lymphatic flow and push the toxins out of the body.

If you are wondering whether your lymphatic function might be compromised, here are some symptoms that could be an indication:

Frequent colds and viral infections

Sinus infections

Swollen glands including tonsils

Lymphedema (swelling in arms or legs)

Frequent headaches

Excess weight

Digestive disorders

Chronic fatigue

How Can You Improve Lymphatic Flow:

There are some simple strategies for supporting your lymphatic system that can be easily, inexpensively and immediately incorporated into your daily routine.

Exercise: Let's begin with exercise and movement. Anything that gets your body moving is great. The most stimulating exercise for the lymphatic system is rebounding on a small trampoline. Rebounding is easy for just about anyone to incorporate, can be high or low intensity and is easy on joints. According to a study done by NASA in 1979, exercising on a trampoline is 68% more efficient than jogging, and an hour of rebounding burns more calories than an hour of jogging. However whatever exercise you choose will get lymph flowing.

<u>Hydration</u>: As I recommend for overall health and for weight loss in **Today is Still the Day**, drink half your body weight in ounces of water per day to further cleanse your system of toxins. Including lemon water is also helpful.

<u>Showers</u>: You can also alternate between hot and cold showers. The hot water dilates the blood vessels, while the cold water shrinks them, which creates a "pump" action that forces lymph to flow. *If you are pregnant or have cardiovascular disease, you are cautioned to avoid this.

<u>Dry Brushing</u>: You can brush your dry skin in a circular motion for 10 minutes by using a natural bristle brush, and then take a shower. Combining this with hot and cold showers increases the benefit.

<u>Deep Breathing</u>: The action of deep breathing is also extremely effective in moving lymph fluid throughout your body.

<u>Lymphatic Massage</u>: Certain chiropractors are skilled in performing this type of specialized massage. Also as women's breasts are very high in lymphatic tunnels and stagnation can manifest in the form of tender or

fibrocystic breasts it may be worthwhile learning how to do **lymphatic massage on your breasts.**

<u>Avoid tight clothing</u>: Excessively tight clothing reduces circulation in the lymphatic system and can cause blockages, which can lead to an accumulation of toxins. This is especially important for women who wear bras all day. I never recommend sleeping with your breasts constricted.

<u>Castor Oil Packs</u>: Castor oil packs have been used for many years for numerous applications including to **stimulate lymph drainage.**

Nutritional Strategies:

There are herbs that can help promote lymphatic flow by reducing inflammation and/or acting as a diuretic, including:

Dandelion Leaf (Taraxacum officinale)

Nettle (Urtica Dioica)

Parsley (Petroselinum crispum)

Lemon peel (Citrus limon L. Osbeck)

Ginger (Zingiber officinale)

Cleavers (Galium aparine)

Calendula (Calendula officinalis)

Red Clover (Trifolium Pratense)

Burdock root (Arctium Lappa)

Eating a diet rich in fresh, whole, nutrient-dense foods will support a healthy lymphatic system. Some cleansing foods for the lymphatic system include:

Leafy green vegetables

Low sugar fruits like berries, apples

Ground flaxseed

Chia seeds

Avocados

Garlic

Brazil nuts

Almonds

Walnuts

Cranberries

Just as important as what foods to eat, are which ones to avoid, and those include:

Processed, packaged foods

Conventionally raised meat, dairy

Artificial sweeteners

Sugar

Soy

Table salt

To simplify, the same foods that support overall health and wellness also support a healthy lymphatic system.

VAGUS NERVE

You may not be familiar with this term so I just wanted to give you a brief overview of what it is and what it does and then talk more specifically about how it impacts immune function in light of where the world is right now. There are actually two parts to the vagus nerve even though it is usually referred to in the singular. It originates in the brain-stem.

The vagus is the 10th of our twelve cranial nerves, which is responsible for parasympathetic control of the heart, lungs and digestion. It is the longest nerve of your autonomic nervous system and the only cranial nerve that leaves the cranial cavity and goes into the rest of the body. By the way the term "vagus" comes from the word wandering because it travels into so many areas of the body.

It activates the parasympathetic nervous system and is essentially our "stress-reset button," having the important job of telling the body that everything is okay.

Let's Talk About the Nervous System:

The nervous system has two parts, the central nervous system (CNS) which is the brain and spinal cord. The peripheral nervous system (PNS) has 2 branches – the somatic which controls voluntary muscle systems and the autonomic, which takes care of those functions like breathing and heart beat that you don't have to consciously control.

The autonomic is further divided into sympathetic (the arousal, fight or flight system) and the parasympathetic (calming, rest and digest system). The parasympathetic fibers of the vagus nerve connect to all organs from the neck to the colon, except the adrenal glands. It is the primary driver of parasympathetic nervous system. It is key in functions like heart rate, breathing rate, peristalsis, sweating, detox and more. It also controls muscles involved in swallowing and speech.

Vagal tone affects our organ systems in profound ways including decreasing heart rate and lowering blood pressure, increasing stomach acid and gastric juices for more effective digestion, suppressing inflammation, keeping anxiety and depression at bay by opposing the sympathetic stress response.

The Polyvagal Theory:

Dr. Stephen Porges **developed this theory that explains our response to stress or danger. The vagus nerve is further divided into 2 branches, the Dorsal Vagus Complex (DVC) which is the more primitive, unmyelinated branch, which is responsible for the freeze response. The Ventral Vagus Complex (VVC), the newer, myelinated branch known as the social engagement system. Activation of the DVC causes immobilization or freeze**

response and activating the VVC causes relaxation and social engagement and the sympathetic fight or flight response.

In a nutshell when the parasympathetic nervous system is functioning properly we are engaged, connected, grounded, mindful and compassionate. This is our rest and digest response. When the sympathetic nervous system is activated we can experience fear, panic, anxiety, anger, frustration, worry, irritation and the impulse to run. This is when adrenaline is released for fight or flight. Then if the DVC branch of the sympathetic system is activated we are immobilized, frozen, numb, depressed.

The sympathetic nervous system is activated in response to stress and affects just about every organ in the body. The fight or flight response is meant to keep us alive. However, when the sympathetic nervous system is in overdrive from chronic stress, as it has been during this health crisis, and emotionally we begin to feel there is no "escape", then the DVC takes over and causes us to shut down or freeze as a form of self-preservation. Our nervous system perceives "danger" even when there is no real, physical threat.

Because even in the best of times most people spend their days in a state of constant, chronic stress, the relaxation response, which should kick in after the threat is over, gets stuck. Sympathetic dominance weakens the rest and digest, detox and heal response and many can no longer effectively activate it when they need to. Another thing to keep in mind is how EMFs are affecting all of us. There is definitely correlation to the vagus nerve which I spoke a bit more about in the section on EMFs.

I compare it to the gas and brake in your car. If you put a brick on your gas pedal while you are in park, your motor would be revving and sooner or later you'd run out of gas. The sympathetic system is the gas pedal for when we need it and the parasympathetic is the brake which helps us calm down and rest.

This is super important to realize: no healing or regeneration takes place during fight, flight or freeze activation. Those systems are focused on survival and healing takes a backseat. We can only heal when the VVC, the relaxation response, is activated.

What Does This Mean for Immune Function:

The bulk of your immune system is in the gut. Studies show gut microorganisms can activate the vagus nerve, which then affects the brain, mood and behavior. Our mind (thoughts, beliefs, emotions) affect gut health and the microbiome (good bacteria) via the vagus nerve. Studies have shown that stress inhibits signals sent through the vagus nerve causing digestive problems. The vagus nerve is a connector between brain and immune system.

The gut-brain axis describes the communication network connecting the gut and the brain with the vagus nerve being a key component. The vagus nerve transmits information in both directions – from brain to gut and from gut to brain. When it is functioning properly, the vagus signals the **shutting down of inflamma-**

tion, which has been associated as the underlying root cause of just about every chronic disease. Chronic inflammation is the most common sign of poor vagal tone. So when inflammation is constant and chronic it keeps the immune response overworked and over time this leads to breakdown of the body.

How Do You Know If Your Vagal Tone is Low:

If you are chronically stressed, chances are very great that your vagal function is compromised. Additionally, if you suffer from any one of these conditions, vagal tone is likely low:

Chronic Fatigue Syndrome

Fibromyalgia

Alzheimers

Parkinson's Disease

Depression, anxiety

Heart disease

Diabetes

Migraines

Autoimmune disease (MS, RA, Lupus, etc.)

Obesity

Cancer

IBS, SIBO, leaky gut

Early life stress/trauma

Negative beliefs

Some other things that indicate low vagal tone include:

Loss of voice or difficulty speaking

Hoarse, wheezy voice

Loss of gag reflex

Trouble drinking liquids

Abnormal heart rate and/or blood pressure

Abdominal bloating, pain

Decreased stomach acid, digestive enzymes

Diarrhea or constipation

The best way to measure whether you have low vagal tone is to measure both resting heart rate and heart rate variability (HRV). Optimal resting heart rate is between 50-70 beats per minute. Heart rate variability is a slight decrease in heart rate with exhalation. Greater heart rate variability (higher vagal tone) is associated with better health including better digestion, reduced inflammation, increased emotional resilience, and longevity. HeartMath Institute has information and techniques for assessing HRV. Interestingly, intermittent fasting, which I covered earlier, has been shown to improve HRV.

Ways to Increase Vagal Tone:

Deep breathing, particularly with long exhalations

Singing, humming, chanting

Yoga, tai chi

Essential oils

Gargling/gag reflex*

Cold showers, and just ending your shower with a blast of cold water

Fasting and intermittent fasting

Probiotics, EFAs, **keeping microbiome healthy**

Eating bitter foods, herbs

Prayer, faith, meditation

EFT

Positive social connection

Expressing gratitude

Laughter, smiling

Biofeedback

*I typically scrape my tongue in the morning before brushing my teeth and intentionally go back far enough on my tongue to stimulate the gag reflex for this purpose. Simply by gargling deeply for 30 seconds a day, is another good way to increase vagal tone.

**Another interesting thing I learned was a bowel transit test since the vagus nerve connects the brain, immune and digestive systems. This doctor suggested mixing 1 tsp. to 1 tbsp. of whole, white sesame seeds in about an ounce of water and drinking it down. Mark down the time you ingest it. Note how long before you first see the sesame seeds in your stool and note that time. Then note when you see them for the last time and note that time. Optimal bowel transit time is 16 hours - but between 12 and 24 is good. If you see them in less than 12 hours or it takes more than 24 then it's a clue that perhaps you could improve vagal tone, which impacts digestion.

Zinc and Quercetin

Zinc is a trace mineral that is essential for regulating the immune system. It helps stimulate the activity of 100 different enzymes and only a very small amount is needed. It's especially vital for a robust immune system by regulating immune response and attacking invading cells, for wound healing **by maintaining skin structure and integrity, synthesizing DNA and proper childhood growth.**

In one study zinc lozenges were found to shorten the duration of a cold by up to 40%.

Quercetin is a natural antioxidant flavonoid found in many foods that plays an important role in helping the body combat free radical damage, which is linked to chronic diseases. It is known to reduce **inflammation**, allergy symptoms and blood pressure.

Importance for COVID-19:

Oral zinc supplementation, especially if you're older is strongly recommended. Two often noted early symptoms of COVID-19 — the loss of taste and smell — are both symptoms of zinc deficiency.

According to this review of COVID19 research, zinc plays a crucial role in the function of essentially all immune cells, and deficiency has a profound impact on immune response, increasing susceptibility to a variety of infections.

Three of the most critical actions of quercetin are that it:

Binds to the **virus responsible for severe acute respiratory syndrome or SARS**, thereby inhibiting its ability to infect host cells.

Acts as a zinc ionophore, which is a compound that shuttles zinc into your cells, one of the mechanisms that can account for the effectiveness seen with hydroxychloroquine, which is also a zinc ionophore.

Quercetin's antiviral capacity is attributed to its ability to inhibit the virus's ability to infect cells, inhibit the replication of infected cells and reduce infected cells' resistance to treatment with antivirals.

Secrets and Tips:

Combining zinc, quercetin and vitamin C seems to be a safe and effective way to approach protecting yourself against COVID 19 as well and other infectious viruses.

However, in order to get the optimal benefit from this strategy it is recommended that it be administered as early in the disease phase as possible. Using quercetin and zinc would be best done if you were recently exposed to the virus in order to inhibit viral replication and keep the viral load low while your immune system does its work in clearing the virus.

It is also recommended that quercetin be taken with liposomal form of vitamin C and zinc in the evening before bed while you are "fasting." This increases your body's ability to recycle quercetin. The other benefit of taking quercetin at night is to take advantage of its senolytic action to remove senescent (aging) cells, which are similar to nonreplicating cancer cells that secrete powerful pro-inflammatory cytokines damaging to your health.

You can optimize quercetin's senolytic properties if you take it while you are fasting. The easiest way for most people to do this is to take it 3 or 4 hours after your last evening meal before sleep.

Foods with the highest reported zinc content are:

raw oysters (Pacific), 3 ounces: 14.1 milligrams

beef, lean chuck roast, braised, 3 ounces: 7.0 milligrams

baked beans, canned, ½ cup: 6.9 milligrams

crab, King Alaskan, cooked, 3 ounces: 6.5 milligrams

ground beef, lean, 3 ounces: 5.3 milligrams

lobster, cooked, 3 ounces: 3.4 milligrams

pork loin, lean, cooked, 3 ounces: 2.9 milligrams

wild rice, cooked, ½ cup: 2.2 milligrams

peas, green, cooked, 1 cup: 1.2 milligrams

yogurt, plain, 8 ounces: 1.3 milligrams

pecans, 1 ounces: 1.3 milligrams

peanuts, dry roasted, 1 ounces: 0.9 milligrams

Vegetarians may require up to 50% more than the recommended intake of zinc because of low bioavailability of zinc from plant-based foods.

Good quercetin food sources include:

capers, peppers

yellow and green onions

red and white shallots

asparagus, cooked

cherries

tomatoes

red apples

red grapes

broccoli

kale, red

leaf lettuce

berries of all types, including cranberries, blueberries, and raspberries and tea — green and black

More Tips

Quercetin is poorly absorbed **by the body which is why it is recommended it be taken with vitamin C. Other research indicates that quercetin has a synergistic effect when combined with other flavonoid supplements, such as resveratrol, genistein, and catechins.**

Products: *indicates product I sell and will receive a commission on.

Zinc + Immune Support lozenges*

Seasonal Immune Support Pack*

Nature's Pearl Muscadine Grape Seed (source of quercetin)*

Metaboblic Flexibility

Last year I did an entire newsletter explaining what metabolic flexibility is, why it is important

for overall health and weight loss and also gave some simple ways to improve your metabolic flexibility. You can read that newsletter right here **and refresh your memory on what it is.**

There is simple and practical information for why this is such an important function. It is especially relevant right now as even mild obesity is known to raise the risk of serious side effects of COVID-19, which of course is top of mind. I am revisiting this because of recent information on how metabolic flexibility plays a role in better COVID-19 outcomes.

Why it's Important:

According to the following criteria used to define metabolic syndrome, it is estimated that at least **9 in 10 Americans are metabolically unhealthy:**

waist circumference of less than 102 cm. (40") for men or 88 cm. (34.6") for women

fasting glucose of less than 100 milligrams per deciliter

hemoglobin A1c of less than 5.7

systolic blood pressure less than 120 and diastolic blood pressure less than 80

triglycerides less than 150

HDL of greater than 40 for men and 50 for women.

As of 2016, 39.8% of adults over the age of 20 were obese. Including those who are overweight increases that percentage to 71%. I've already done a newsletter on how excess weight typically correlates with metabolic dysfunction and impaired health as well as how they impact immune function.

How do you stack up when considering these criteria? It may be wise to assess where you stand right now and what you may need to improve. One of the most common changes associated with insulin resistance, obesity and metabolic syndrome is over-activation of the innate immune system, with decreasing activity in the adaptive immune system.

It may be helpful here to give a quick explanation on the two arms of your immune system to better understand why this is so critical.

The Innate Immune System:

This is the part that we as individuals can either fortify or destroy by our daily habits and lifestyle. It is the first part of the immune system to the fight when we are exposed to a pathogen. The innate immune system includes various types of white blood cells like phagocytes (macrophages, mast cells, etc.) and monocytes, the various neutrophils (like eosinophils, basophils, natural killer cells) that destroy infected host cells, as well as another kind of neutrophil called dendritic cells.

Then there are various proteins released by these cells, that act as cell signaling messengers coordinating the attack on an invader. All of them team up to destroy, engulf or digest the foreign or pathogenic invader. B cells and T (Thymus) cells, which are both lymphocytes, have several important roles within the innate immune system. Some of these cells are also involved in the activation of the second arm of the immune system, the adaptive immune system.

The Adaptive Immune System:

This kicks in a few days after the infection begins producing antibodies to join the fight. It is truly remarkable how God created our bodies to respond and how all of this is orchestrated! If at a later date the person is exposed to the same virus, the adaptive immune system will recognize that virus and produce antibodies to help the innate immune system fend off that specific attacker. Although this part of the immune system is not influenced by lifestyle, diet and supplementation to the same degree as the Innate immune system, those lifestyle components are still influential.

So when it comes to healthy aging, your biological age matters less than your immune and metabolic age, both of which can be improved through simple lifestyle changes. *The good news is that there are many things you can do to change your susceptibility to this virus, if you are willing to make some changes.*

So, in a nutshell, when blood sugar is well-controlled and there's less glycemic variability, people do better when contracting COVID-19. When they have high levels of glycemic variability, which indicates insulin resistance, they fare much worse.

Another Interesting Factor:

Mainstream medicine pushes statins to get LDL cholesterol and total cholesterol as low as possible. Research shows that low levels of LDL cholesterol are associated with greater COVID-19 severity. LDL and total cholesterol levels were significantly lower in COVID-19 patients as compared to healthy subjects.

Cholesterol, contained in this LDL lipoprotein parti-cle, is intimately involved in the immune response. In someone who is metabolically healthy, a higher LDL above 100 or 150, or even 200 mg/dL might not be the horrible thing that we've all been taught it is, particu-larly if the HDL, triglycerides, **triglyceride to glucose index (TyG index)**, and glycemic variability, are all in-dicating metabolic health.

So What Can You Do?

My first recommendation, regardless of the prob-lem, is **nutrition**. Eating high quality, properly raised/ grown, real, whole, one-ingredient foods. As I have said numerous times that means organic, grass-fed and finished and pasture raised. It also means elimi-nating packaged, processed, junk foods, gluten, grains, processed carbs, sugar and vegetable oils. Let me sug-gest here that you consider including or reintroducing properly raised animal foods as many nutrient deficien-cies that affect immune function come primarily from animal foods.

Try implementing **intermittent fasting**. Another powerful strategy to improve insulin sensitivity is by compressing the window of time in which you eat down to six to eight hours a day and eating your last meal at least three hours before bedtime. This is a form of intermittent fasting.

You have a 6 or 8 hour window during which you eat your meals and then fast the remaining 16 or 18 hours (most of which you are sleeping). I do this most days of the week and it is a powerful strategy. It is not nearly as difficult as you may be thinking and I explained a bit more about it at the beginning and in **Today is Still The Day**. Intermittent fasting or time-restricted eating allows you to become metabolically flexible and insulin sensitive, which builds your antifragility.

I hope you come away with the understanding that there are things you can do to improve your overall health as well as your immune function. If you need more help with this, please don't hesitate to request a consultation or click this link and schedule a zoom, skype or phone call.

Here are links to products and also blogs, newsletters and articles mentioned in the book in case you have the paperback version:

Pique tea https://www.piquetea.com/

***Today is Still the Day** https://amzn.to/2DJAM-IX

Masaru Emoto https://www.masaru-emoto.net/en/crystal/

***Youngevity Super Greens** https://3dlivingnutrition.youngevity.com/us_en/catalog/product/view/id/953

OrganiGreens

https://shop.organixx.com/collections/all-products/products/organigreens

Bone Broth https://www.vitacost.com/om-mushroom-mighty-beef-bone-broth-drink-mix

Collagen Broth https://drkellyann.com/products/collagen-broth?variant=30992101898

Coconut Oil https://www.vitacost.com/vita-cost-certified-organic-unrefined-coconut-oil

Manuka Honey https://www.swansonvitamins.com/wedderspoon-raw-manuka-honey-kfactor-16-17-6-oz-500-grams-jar

Flax Seeds https://www.vitacost.com/barleans-organic-forti-flax?ta=Barleans+ground+flax-+seeds&t=Barleans+ground+flax+seeds

Beef Sticks https://paleovalley.com/store/beef-sticks

Turkey Sticks https://paleovalley.com/store/pasture-raised-turkey-sticks

*Youngevity Collagen Peptides https://3dliving-nutrition.youngevity.com/us_en/collagen-pep-tides.html

*Slender FX Meal Replacement Shake https://3dlivingnutrition.youngevity.com/us_en/food-beverage/shakes/meal-replacement/slender-fx-meal-replacement-shake-chocolate-fudge-384.html

*TMR Total Meal Replacement Shake https://3dlivingnutrition.youngevity.com/us_en/food-beverage/shakes/meal-replacement/tmr-total-meal-replacement-shake-30-day.html

*Youngevity FitShake https://3dlivingnutrition.youngevity.com/us_en/food-beverage/shakes/performance/youngevity-fitshake-trade.html

*Slender FX True Keto Shake https://3dlivingnutrition.youngevity.com/us_en/food-beverage/shakes/weight-management/trueketo-shake.html

NOW Vitamin C https://www.vitacost.com/now-foods-c-1000-500-veg-capsules?ta=NOW+Foods+Vitamin+C&t=now+foods+vitamin+c

Vitamin D3 https://www.vitacost.com/vitacost-vitamin-d3-as-cholecalciferol-2000-iu-120-softgels-minigels

*Ultimate Selenium https://3dlivingnutrition.youngevity.com/us_en/catalog/product/view/id/6752/s/ultimate-selenium-778/category/1268/

Quercetin https://www.ncbi.nlm.nih.gov/pmc/articles/PMC4808895/

Zinc Lozenges https://www.swansonvitamins.com/natures-way-zinc-60-lozenges

Manuka Honey Drops with Bee Propolis https://www.swansonvitamins.com/wedderspoon-organic-manuka-honey-drops-lemon-bee-propolis-4-oz-120-grams-pkg

Melatonin https://www.swansonvitamins.com/q?kw=melatonin

Tryptophan https://www.swansonvitamins.com/now-foods-l-tryptophan-500-mg-120-vcaps

Research re Melatonin https://articles.mercola.com/sites/articles/archive/2020/04/02/melatonin-and-sepsis.aspx?cid_source=dnl&cid_medium=email&cid_content=art1HL&cid=20200402Z1&et_cid=DM495138&et_rid=842558233

Vitacost Probiotic https://www.vitacost.com/vitacost-probiotic-15-35-15-strains-35-billion-cfu-per-serving-120-vegetarian-capsules

Organixx Probiotixx https://shop.organixx.com/collections/all-products/products/probiotixx

Just Thrive Probiotic https://justthrivehealth.com/

Organixx P3E https://shop.organixx.com/products/p3e

R-Garden Protease https://www.rgarden.com/protease.html

*Ultimate Colloidal Silver Plus https://3dlivingnutrition.youngevity.com/us_en/catalog/product/view/id/586/category/1268/

Vitacost Kelp https://www.vitacost.com/vitacost-kelp

Survival Shield X-2 Nascent Iodine https://www.infowarsstore.com/survival-shield-x-2-nascent-iodine?gclid=CjwKCAjw3-bzBRBhEiwAgnnLClh-qh-6PpnpUP9zSjT9DbtPmRh9VQWtEFyxfyLzdy-QgU_Izr-7vgoBoCO-UQAvD_BwE

*RVB 300 (BetaGlucan) https://3dlivingnutrition.youngevity.com/us_en/catalog/product/view/id/621/category/1268/

NAC https://www.vitacost.com/vitacost-n-acetyl-l-cysteine-600-mg-240-capsules

Crucial Role of NAC in Preventing COVID https://articles.mercola.com/sites/articles/archive/2020/11/10/coronavirus-n-acetylcysteine.aspx?cid_source=dnl&cid_medium=email&cid_content=art1HL&cid=20201110Z1&mid=DM706746&rid=1007979644

OM Immune Mushroom Powder https://www.swansonvitamins.com/mushroom-matrix-immuneog1powder200grm-7-14-oz-7-14-oz

Lauricidin https://www.lauricidin.com/

Senolytic Activator https://www.lifeextension.com/vitamins-supplements/item02301/senolytic-activator

Wholetones https://wholetones.com/

Health and Longevity: More Gratitude Benefits https://amusico.wordpress.com/2014/12/01/health-and-longevity-more-gratitude-benefits-that-may-surprise-you/

Brain Health: Why Gratitude is Powerful https://amusico.wordpress.com/2016/07/18/brain-health-why-gratitude-is-powerful/

Health Benefits of Gratitude https://amusico.wordpress.com/2019/11/25/health-benefits-of-gratitude/

The Good Old Days Exercise https://www.threedimensionalvitality.com/good_old_days_exercise.html

Health and Stress: Nature is a Natural Stress Reducer and Productivity Booster https://amusico.wordpress.com/2015/11/30/health-and-stress-nature-is-a-natural-stress-reducer-and-productivity-booster/

Health and Wholeness: Getting Back to Nature https://amusico.wordpress.com/2016/09/26/health-and-wholeness-getting-back-to-nature/

Health: The Nature Prescription https://amusico.wordpress.com/2018/09/24/healthy-the-nature-prescription/

Health and Emotions: We Can't Overlook Their Impact on Health Part 2 https://amusico.wordpress.com/2015/11/02/health-and-emotions-we-cant-overlook-their-impact-on-health-part-two/

Obesity https://www.webmd.com/lung/news/20200416/obesity-link-to-severe-covid-19-especially-in-the-under-60s?src=RSS_PUBLIC#1

Obesity, Coronavirus and Younger People https://www.nytimes.com/2020/04/16/health/coronavirus-obesity-higher-risk.html

Insulin Resistance https://articles.mercola.com/sites/articles/archive/2020/05/04/insulin-resistance-the-real-pandemic.aspx?cid_source=dnl&cid_medium=email&cid_content=art1HL&cid=20200504Z1&et_cid=DM527834&et_rid=864587365

Diabetes and COVID https://articles.mercola.com/sites/articles/archive/2020/04/30/blood-sugar-rising.aspx?cid_source=dnl&cid_medium=email&cid_content=art1HL&cid=20200430Z1&et_cid=DM521283&et_rid=861823375

Today is Still the Day 7 Week Coaching Plan https://www.threedimensionalvitality.com/3_D_Weight_Loss_Plan.html

Impact of Obesity on Immune Function https://www.longdom.org/open-access/the-impact-of-obesity-on-immune-response-to-infection-and-vaccine-an-insight-into-plausible-mechanisms-2161-1017.1000113.pdf

Infections and Diabetes https://www.ncbi.nlm.nih.gov/pmc/articles/PMC3354930/

High Blood Sugar and Immune System Malfunction https://www.sciencedaily.com/releases/2015/08/150806151354.htm

Better Oral Health Can Boost Immune Function https://drania.com/better-oral-health-can-boost-your-immune-system/

Diabetes and Oral Health https://www.nidcr.nih.gov/health-info/diabetes

Foods for Oral Health http://hosted.vresp.com/503323/0e26d58a5f/1503001362/51908a8c3f/

Sleep Habits and Susceptibility to Common Cold https://www.ncbi.nlm.nih.gov/pmc/articles/PMC2629403/

Chiropractic Study https://www.summitfamilychiropractictn.com/blog/chiropractic-immunity-boost#:~:text=The%20chiropractic%20patients%20were%20found,cancer%20and%20other%20serious%20diseases.

Free Consultation https://www.threedimensionalvitality.com/free-phone-consultation.html

Ultra Processed Food Dangers

https://articles.mercola.com/sites/articles/archive/2020/04/29/ultraprocessed-food-makes-you-vulnerable-to-covid-19.aspx?cid_source=dnl&cid_medium=email&cid_content=art2HL&cid=20200429Z1&et_cid=DM521251&et_rid=861065477

What is Nutrient Density https://chriskresser.com/what-is-nutrient-density-and-why-is-it-important/

Intermittent Fasting and Inflammation https://pubmed.ncbi.nlm.nih.gov/23244540/

Interlukin 6, C Reactive Protein and Intermittent Fasting https://pubmed.ncbi.nlm.nih.gov/17374948/

Earthing https://www.ncbi.nlm.nih.gov/pmc/articles/PMC3265077/

Effects of Grounding on Inflammation https://www.ncbi.nlm.nih.gov/pmc/articles/PMC4378297/

Health Benefit of Exercise https://pubmed.ncbi.nlm.nih.gov/32220789/

Exercise May Protect Against ARDS https://www.eurekalert.org/pub_releases/2020-04/uovh-cem041520.php

Exercise and The Immune System During Aging https://www.mdpi.com/2072-6643/12/3/622/htm

Health Effects of Chronic Fear https://www.ajmc.com/view/the-effects-of-chronic-fear-on-a-persons-health

Psychological Factors Influencing Health https://pubmed.ncbi.nlm.nih.gov/6701256/

Healthy Lifestyle and Psychological Health Link https://www.ncbi.nlm.nih.gov/pmc/articles/PMC5387968/

Mood and Cytokine Response to Flu in Older Adults https://pubmed.ncbi.nlm.nih.gov/15699534/

Positive Emotions and Resistance to Illness https://pubmed.ncbi.nlm.nih.gov/17101814/

Psychological well-being and Sleep https://pubmed.ncbi.nlm.nih.gov/18374740/

Emotional Style and Susceptibility to Common Cold https://pubmed.ncbi.nlm.nih.gov/12883117/

Fighting COVID with Water https://articles.mercola.com/sites/articles/archive/2020/05/11/can-humidity-help-fight-against-covid-19.aspx?cid_source=dnl&cid_medium=email&cid_content=art3HL&cid=20200511Z1&et_cid=DM534048&et_rid=869393315

Relative Indoor Humidity and Health https://www.ncbi.nlm.nih.gov/pmc/articles/PMC1474709/

Indoor Transmission of SARS COV-2 https://www.medrxiv.org/content/medrxiv/early/2020/04/07/2020.04.04.20053058.full.pdf

Humidity as an Intervention for Flu https://journals.plos.org/plosone/article?id=10.1371/journal.pone.0204337

Voltage-Gated Calcium Channel Activation https://pubmed.ncbi.nlm.nih.gov/25879308/

5G Fact Sheet https://www.telecompowergrab.org/uploads/3/8/5/9/38599771/5g_fact_sheet_v9.pdf

EMFs and Suppressed Immune Function https://pubmed.ncbi.nlm.nih.gov/11855293/

Active Denial System FAQs https://jnlwp.defense.gov/About/Frequently-Asked-Questions/Active-Denial-System-FAQs/

5G Human Health Risks https://ehtrust.org/key-issues/cell-phoneswireless/5g-networks-iot-scientific-overview-human-health-risks/

5G and COVID https://www.5gspaceappeal.org/the-appeal

Association between COVID Cases and 5G https://magdahavas.com/5g-and-mm-waves/is-there-an-association-between-covid-19-cases-deaths-and-5g-in-the-united-states/

Connection between COVID 19 and 5G https://lifeenergysolutions.com/blog/is-there-a-connection-between-covid-19-and-5g/

Faraday Bags https://www.amazon.com/Mission-Darkness-Non-Window-Faraday-Phones/dp/B01A7MACL2

2 page 5G Fact Sheet https://ehtrust.org/wp-content/uploads/5G_What-You-Need-to-Know.pdf

*The Quantum Difference Q3 Bands http://quantum3.life/vibrantlife

Compelling Videos https://thequantumdifference.com/?pdx-ts=1605309129&pdx-sid=de5e2352a-4b62e9329faef4e097fe1b4

Science Behind Q3 Bands http://www.quantumnutritionallife.com/Quantum3-Science

O2 Uptake during Running and Jumping https://pubmed.ncbi.nlm.nih.gov/7429911/

Lymphatic Breast Massage https://www.wellandgood.com/breast-massage-health-benefits-how-to/

Castor Oil Packs for Lymphatic Drainage https://theartofhealingtouch.com/how-to-make-castor-oil-packs-for-lymphatic-drainage/

Stephen Porges Polyvagal Theory https://www.stephenporges.com/bio

Vagus Connects Brain to Immune System https://www.sciencedaily.com/releases/2007/10/071024083630.htm

Vagus Nerve Stimulation https://www.mayoclinic.org/tests-procedures/vagus-nerve-stimulation/about/pac-20384565

Vagus Nerve and Migraines https://www.mayoclinic.org/tests-procedures/vagus-nerve-stimulation/about/pac-20384565

HeartMath https://www.heartmath.org/

Vagus Nerve and Deep Breathing https://www.psychologytoday.com/us/blog/the-athletes-way/201905/longer-exhalations-are-easy-way-hack-your-vagus-nerve

Cold Stimulation for Vagus https://www.ncbi.nlm.nih.gov/pmc/articles/PMC6334714/

Probiotics and Vagus Nerve https://pubmed.ncbi.nlm.nih.gov/21876150/

Vagus as Moderator of Gut-Brain Axis https://www.frontiersin.org/articles/10.3389/fpsyt.2018.00044/full

Prayer https://www.threedimensionalvitality.com/A_Sincere_Invitation.html

EFT https://www.threedimensionalvitality.com/tapping-into-health.html

Zinc and Immune Function https://pubmed.ncbi.nlm.nih.gov/9701160/

Zinc and Wound Healing https://pubmed.ncbi.nlm.nih.gov/2275309/

Zinc Lozenges Shorten Duration of Colds https://www.ncbi.nlm.nih.gov/pmc/articles/PMC3136969/

Health Effects of Quercetin https://pubmed.ncbi.nlm.nih.gov/18417116/

Quercetin and Anti-Allergic Response https://pubmed.ncbi.nlm.nih.gov/27187333/

Zinc and Covid Research https://athmjournal.com/covid19/wp-content/uploads/sites/4/2020/05/imcj-19-08.pdf

SARS https://pubmed.ncbi.nlm.nih.gov/15452254/

Zinc Ionophore Activity of Quercetin and EGCG https://pubs.acs.org/doi/full/10.1021/jf5014633

Quercetin Anti-Viral Activity https://pubmed.ncbi.nlm.nih.gov/20934345/

Bioavailability of Quercetin https://pubmed.ncbi.nlm.nih.gov/28377278/

Quercetin and Vitamin C https://www.frontiersin.org/articles/10.3389/fimmu.2020.01451/full

Improving Bioavailability through Synergy https://pubmed.ncbi.nlm.nih.gov/19841960/

*Zinc Plus Immune Support https://3dlivingnutrition.youngevity.com/us_en/zinc-immune-support.html

*Seasonal Immune Support Pack https://3dlivingnutrition.youngevity.com/us_en/seasonal-immune-support-pak-30ct-967.html

*Premium Muscadine Grape Seed https://3dlivingnutrition.youngevity.com/us_en/buy-1-get-1-premium-muscadine-grape-seed.html

Metabolic Flexibility http://hosted.vresp.com/503323/daf87c302e/1503001362/51908a8c3f/

Metabolic Health in American Adults https://www.liebertpub.com/doi/10.1089/met.2018.0105

Immune and Metabolic Age https://www.nature.com/articles/s41591-019-0381-y

Blood Sugar Control and COVID 19 https://www.sciencedirect.com/science/article/pii/S1550413120302382

Association of Insulin Resistance to COVID Severity and Mortality https://cardiab.biomedcentral.com/articles/10.1186/s12933-020-01035-2

Metabolic Flexibility and Insulin Sensitivity https://articles.mercola.com/sites/articles/archive/2020/08/16/small-stressors-beneficial.aspx?cid_source=dnl&cid_medium=email&cid_content=art2HL&cid=20200816Z1&mid=DM627875&rid=941634516

Embracing Uncertainty https://amusico.wordpress.com/2020/05/18/embracing-uncertainty-perception-truth-and-faith/

Should Masks Continue https://articles.mercola.com/sites/articles/archive/2020/11/14/mandatory-masks.aspx?ui=25cec8f3367f70110f-

7cda162411daa73353c8abf01ca49356413cac9e-9a2043&cid_source=dnl&cid_medium=email&cid_content=art1HL&cid=20201114Z1&mid=D-M706757&rid=1011049718

My Morning Elixir https://www.threedimensionalvitality.com/articles/article/8754673/193539.htm

EGCG in Green Tea benefits Immune Function https://www.japanesegreenteain.com/blogs/green-tea-and-health/how-green-tea-helps-to-improve-your-immune-system

MY PERSONAL PROTOCOL

As I said this is simply what I do and is shared as an example of some things you may want to begin incorporating into your daily routine. We are all unique beings and what works for me may not be right for you.

Upon waking: I scrape my tongue and rinse my mouth before eating or drinking anything. I usually scrape 3 or 4 times, with at least 2 to the point of gagging to engage the vagus nerve.

I practice intermittent fasting most days of the week, usually either 16-8 or 18-6 so before I have my **morning elixir** which includes both green and black tea as well as mushroom coffee, all of which have health and immune benefits, I have 16 oz of water with ½ tsp of natural, unprocessed Himalayan Crystal Salt and my probiotic. This is the first part of my one-half my body weight in ounces, not counting teas.

I spend time in prayer and journaling. Stress and anxiety, especially at this time are as serious a risk factor to contracting COVID or any other illness as what you eat and drink. I also take communion daily. I use EFT whenever I feel myself getting stressed or anxious and

I try to do it in the moment, when I feel those emotions, as much as I am able.

My morning elixir, which I usually have around 8 am serves as my breakfast.

Before I floss and brush my teeth for the morning, I typically oil pull. I shoot for at least 3 or 4 days out of the week depending on how busy the morning is. This is a powerful way to detox not only for oral health but also for immune health as I mentioned earlier.

As for my usual supplements, I take 3-4,000 IU of vitamin C daily normally, 5,000 IU of vitamin D3, 600 mg of NAC, at least 400 mg of magnesium depending on the source (whether glycinate or threonate); black garlic and the rest of my daily supplements.

On Monday mornings I include a sachet of Pique Pu'ehr and/or Reishi tea in my morning elixir and on Monday evenings both my husband and I take the Senolytic Activator before bed on an empty stomach. That supplement only needs to be taken once a week.

If I feel a bit under the weather, haven't gotten enough sleep or I have been around a lot of people and want extra protection, I take quercetin, vitamin A, zinc, resveratrol, liposomal vitamin C and I take them at night, before bed, during my fasting window to reap the greatest benefit from them. I would do this for a couple of days. I would also use zinc lozenges several times a day.

Another thing I do, immediately, if I feel like I am starting to get a scratchy throat or just feel under the weather is to take protease enzyme at night during my fasting window in order for it to have the opportunity to scavenge any viruses or bacteria. I would do this for a few days as well.

I wear my **Q3 band** daily to keep my cells open to nutrition and to be as protected as possible from EMF exposure.

I exercise 5 or 6 days a week. When weather permits I walk outside in the sunshine and fresh air which boost health, and I try to get at least 7 hours of deep, rejuvenating sleep daily.

I eat fresh, whole, one-ingredient foods at least 90% of the time. I restrict sugar, grains and processed foods and am mindful of keeping my glucose levels steady in order to avoid developing insulin resistance. I regularly include bone broth and fermented foods like miso, sauerkraut and kimchi as well as taking a daily probiotic. In the warmer months I also enjoy kombucha.

As I said, this is just what I do and is offered as an example that you can use to structure your own personal protocol. It is not intended as a specific recommendation. ***Always check with your own healthcare provider before making any changes.***

My prayer is that you have found some information that will be useful in keeping you and your family healthy.

I invite you to visit my website: https://www.threedimensionalvitality.com or www.annmusico.com

There are many free resources there and you can sign up for a free consultation. If you have any questions email me at ann@threedimensionalvitality.com

Health and Blessings,

Ann